THE ANTI-INFLAMMATORY COOKBOOK FOR YOU AND YOUR FAMILY

50 Recipes Easy Medically Accurate to Prepare and to Stay Healthy

Artsy Chef

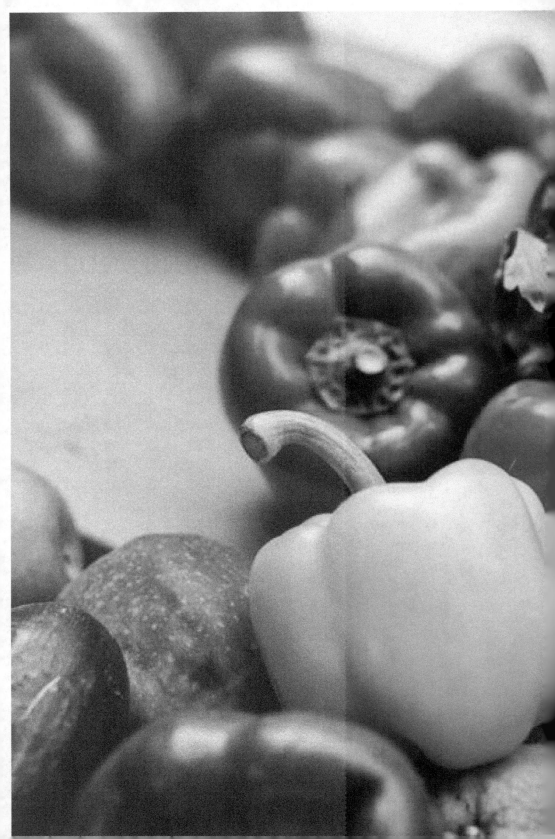

Table of Contents

INTRODUCTION

The anti-inflammatory diet is the best diet for conditions that cause inflammation such as asthma, chronic peptic ulcer, tuberculosis, rheumatoid arthritis, period on it is Crohn's disease, sinusitis, active hepatitis, etc. Along with medical treatment, proper nutrition is very important. An anti-inflammatory diet can help to reduce the pain from inflammation and supplement other treatments.

Inflammation is a natural response of your body to infections, injuries, and illnesses. The classic symptoms are redness, pain, heat, and swelling. Nevertheless, some diseases such as diabetes, heart disease, and cancer produce no symptoms. An anti-inflammatory diet is a great preventive way to safeguard your health.

The anti-inflammatory diet provides antioxidants and reduces the level of free radicals in our bodies. The most common question that people ask is what to eat while on the anti-inflammatory diet. Recommended foods are fruit, vegetables, whole grains, plant-based proteins, and fish, as well as spices, condiments, and dressings. The only condition that should be followed is that all food should be organic.

The most popular vegetables and fruits for the diet are leafy greens, cherries, raspberries, blackberries, tomatoes, cucumbers, etc. Grains include oatmeal, brown rice, and all grains that are high in fiber. Herbs and spices are natural antioxidants that will boost your health as they add flavor. You should avoid highly processed food such as sugary drinks, chocolate, ice cream, French fries, burgers, sausages, deli meats, and overly greasy food. One more factor that will help is making sure you get enough water per day. It is easy to track. There are a lot of apps that will help you to do it correctly. Drinking plenty of water helps the body to cleanse faster.

The anti-inflammatory diet is simple to follow and is not restrictive. There are many ways to adjust it to your preferences. Nevertheless, there are some cons that you should know. It can be costly since it recommends eating all organic food. It also contains a lot of allergens such as nuts, seeds, and soy.

However, eating the right adjusted food will help to eliminate the cons of the diet. It is highly recommended to go to your doctor for a complete medical examination before starting the diet.

This is important information that you should know before starting any diet. A diet is not a magic remedy for all diseases, but it does support the body in conjunction with treatment. Start your new healthy life with one small step, and you will see huge results within half a year. You can be sure that your body will respond by giving you a fresh look and energy for new achievements.

What to Eat and Avoid on the Anti-Inflammatory Diet

- **Meat, Poultry, and Fish**

The best choice for an anti-inflammatory diet is fish and seafood. This type of food is rich in omega-3 fatty acids. Meat can be eaten in moderation, although it is recommended to eat grass-fed meat.

What to eat	Eat occasionally	What to avoid
Tuna	Beef	Lamb
Sole	Chicken	Lard
Shrimps	Pork loin	Bacon
Turkey	Pork tenderloin	pork
Halibut		Breaded fish
Trout		
Salmon		
Flounder		

Mackerel		
Oysters		
Sardines		
Catfish		
Clams		
Cod		
Crab		
Herring		

- **Dairy**

Dairy products can be both useful and harmful to your health. Full-fat dairy products can cause acne and increase inflammatory conditions.

What to eat	Eat occasionally	What to avoid
Non-fat milk	Rice milk	Whole cream
Low-fat milk	Skim milk	Sour cream

Coconut milk	Tofu cheese	Cream
Greek-style yogurt	Parmesan	Hard cheese
Fat-free plain traditional yogurt		Milk butter
		Margarine
Cashew butter		Cottage cheese
Sunflower seeds butter		

- **Eggs**

Eggs contain essential nutrients, proteins, lutein, and zeaxanthin, which all fight inflammation. Nevertheless, frequent consumption of eggs can cause allergic reactions.

- **Nuts and Seeds**

Nuts and seeds are good for heart health. They are rich in fiber and nutrition. Only eat them if you're sure you have no sensitivities.

What to eat	Eat occasionally	What to avoid
Almonds	Hazelnuts	Chocolate-covered nuts
Chia seeds	Cashews	
Flaxseeds	Peanut butter	Nut butter (sweetened/ unsweetened)
Pumpkin seeds		Macadamia nuts
Pistachios		Peanuts
		Pecans

- **Vegetables**

The main source of vitamins during the anti-inflammatory diet is vegetables. However, not all vegetables are beneficial. Avoid starchy vegetables and vegetables that can cause allergic reactions.

What to eat	Eat occasionally	What to avoid
Sweet potatoes	Tomatoes	Potatoes
Yams	Tomatillos	Potato chips
Beets	Corn	Mushrooms
Radishes		
Watermelon		
Green beans		
Organic baked corn chips		
Sweet peppers		
Shiitake mushrooms		
Bell peppers		

- **Fruits and Berries**

Fruits are rich in vitamins. Nevertheless, avoid eating large amounts of sugary fruits. Replace them with sweet and sour or sour fruits/berries.

What to eat	Eat occasionally	What to avoid
Tart cherries	Kiwi	Acerola
Strawberries	Papaya	Lychee
Blueberries	Bananas	Persimmon
Apples		
Pears		
Apricots		
Avocado		
Dried fruits		

Oranges Mangoes Pineapple		

- **Grain Products**

Whole-grains are rich in fiber and can fight inflammation and protect our body from infection. Avoid eating "bad" grains.

What to eat	What to avoid
Brown rice	White rice
Wild rice	Sugar cereals
Oatmeal	White bread
Whole-grain bread	Crackers
Multigrain bread	Snacks
Whole-grain pasta	Rye bread
Oat flour	Wheat noodles
Buckwheat flour	White bread crumbs
Whole wheat flour	Corn flour

Rice noodles	Wheat tortillas
Corn tortillas	Bagels
Whole-grain toast	

- **Condiments**

Condiments play a significant role in flavor. They can make a meal tender, spicy, or salty. On your anti-inflammatory diet, you can use almost all spices and herbs. They have strong anti-inflammatory features.

What to eat	What to avoid
Low-fat mayonnaise	Mayonnaise (full-fat)
Ground pink peppercorns	Tartar sauce
Turmeric tahini dressing	Teriyaki
Alfredo sauce	Tomato sauce
Hot red pepper sauce	Bordelaise sauce
Chimichurri sauce	Brown sauce
Curry powder	Chili sauce
Tapatio sauce (handmade)	Dijon sauce
Apple cider vinegar	Buffalo sauce
Pomegranate sauce	Hollandaise sauce

	Marinara sauce
	Worcestershire sauce
	Sweet and sour sauce
	Soy sauce
	Pickle relish
	Barbecue sauce
	Dijon mustard

- **Oils and fats**

It is recommended to consume vegetable oils and fats during the anti-inflammatory diet. Bear in mind that some natural oils can cause allergies.

What to eat	Eat occasionally	What to avoid
Sunflower oil (cold-pressed) Grapes seed oil	Walnut oil	Coconut oil Palm oil

Olive oil (extra virgin) Flax seeds oil		

- **Beverages**

Drinking water should be a rule for you during the anti-inflammatory diet. Nevertheless, not all drinks are created equal. Avoid consuming sparkling drinks and beverages that contain artificial sugars.

What to eat	Eat occasionally	What to avoid
Fresh fruits	Fresh juice	Coffee
Seltzer		Sodas
Filtered water		Wine
Mineral water		Sparkling mineral water
Lemon water		Carbonated drinks
Herbal tea		Sweet sparkling beverages

Green tea		
Mate tea		

- **Sweets**

Fruits are the best sweets during the anti-inflammatory diet. They are rich in vitamins and contain only natural sweeteners.

Nevertheless, you can find a lot of sugar-free meals which are not inferior in taste to the most famous desserts.

What to eat	Eat occasionally	What to avoid
Honey	Stevia	Artificial sweeteners
Raw cocoa powder	Xylitol	Buns
Fruits (allowed for anti-inflammatory diet)	Brown rice syrup	Candy
	Dark chocolate	Cakes
		Chocolate
		Cookies

		Custard
		Ice cream
		Pastries
		Pies
		Pudding
		Sugar
		Tarts
		Corn syrup
		Milk chocolate

- **Beans and Legumes**

Consumption of beans and legumes is very important during the anti-inflammatory diet. They are rich in fiber and contain large amounts of protein as well as antioxidants. It is necessary to eat at least two servings of beans or legumes per week.

Note that beans and legumes can cause inflammation only if they are cooked in the wrong way. It is recommended to soak beans before cooking.

- **Others**

Fast food and processed food are forbidden during the anti-inflammatory diet. Such food damages our digestive and immune system.

Top 10 Anti-Inflammatory Diet Tips

- **Avoid white food**

Avoiding white food such as sugar, salt, etc. can help to maintain and control the normal level of blood sugar. Try to add more lean proteins and high fiber food to your daily diet. It can be lean types of meat, brown rice, and whole grains.

- **An apple a day keeps the doctors away**

Add vegetables, fruits, nuts, and spices to your daily meal plan. Garlic, ginger, cinnamon, and lemon will help to boost your immune system and reduce inflammation.

- **Exercise daily**

Regular sports activities can help to prevent inflammation. Do 5-10 minutes of exercise daily to feel healthier.

- **Balance your mind**

Everyday stress leads to chronic diseases. Practicing yoga, meditation, or biofeedback are excellent ways to balance your mind and manage stress.

- **Choose the right proteins**

Lean red meat can be served as a source of proteins but it is still high in cholesterol and salt. Instead, choose fish such as halibut, salmon, tuna, cod, or seabass. They are rich in omega-3 fatty acids.

- **Drink antioxidant beverages**

Herbs are a great source of antioxidants and promote faster treatment. Basil, thyme, oregano, chili pepper, and curcumin have high anti-inflammatory features and serve as natural painkillers.

- **Get enough sleep**

You should always get 8-9 hours of sleep at night. Too much or too little sleep is the main triggers for heart disease and type 2 diabetes.

- **Cross out alcohol from your diet**

Avoiding alcohol helps keep you calm and reduces the risk of inflammation.

Choose green tea instead of coffee or black tea.

Green tea can fight free radical damage. Drinking green tea regularly lowers the risk of cancer and Alzheimer's disease.

- **Consume probiotics every day**

Urban lifestyle and junk food is bad for your digestion. Eating food that is rich in probiotics like sauerkraut, yogurt, milk, kombucha, miso, kimchi, and fermented vegetables/fruits every day will improve your gut's microbe barrier.

BREAKFAST

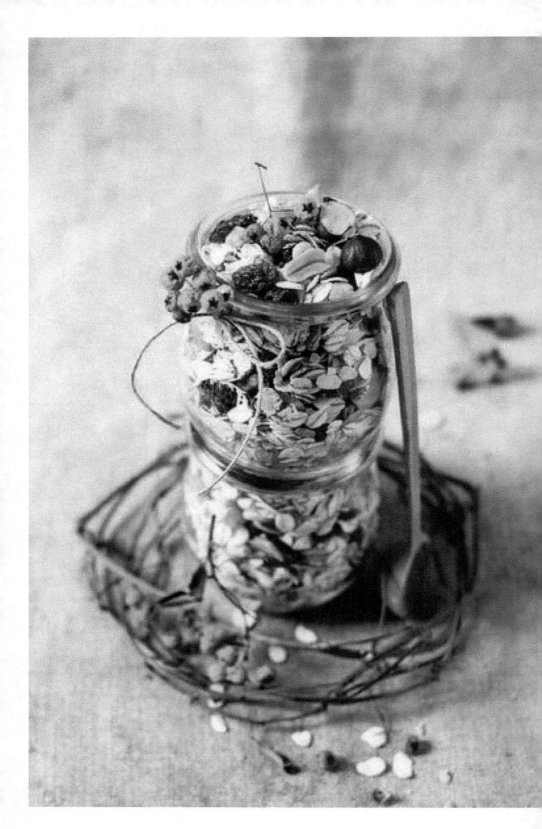

Chia Pudding

2 Servings

Preparation Time: 4 hours

Ingredients

- 2 cups Coconut milk, unsweetened
- 1 Banana, peeled and sliced
- ½ cup chia seeds
- ½ teaspoon Vanilla extract
- 2 tablespoons raw honey
- 1 tablespoon cocoa powder
- 2 tablespoons cocoa nibs

Directions

- In a bowl, mix the Banana with the chia seeds, and mash using a fork.
- Add the milk, the vanilla extract, honey, cocoa powder and cocoa nibs, mix and keep in the fridge for 4 hours before serving.

Pineapple and Orange Smoothie

2 Servings

Preparation Time: 10 minutes

Ingredients

- 1 cup Coconut Water
- 1 orange, peeled and cut into quarters
- 1½ cups Pineapple chunks
- 1 tablespoon fresh grated Ginger
- 1 teaspoon chia seeds
- 1 teaspoon turmeric powder
- A pinch of black pepper

Directions

- In your food processor, mix the Coconut Water with the orange, Pineapple, Ginger, chia seeds, turmeric and black pepper.
- Pulse well, pour into a glass and serve for breakfast.

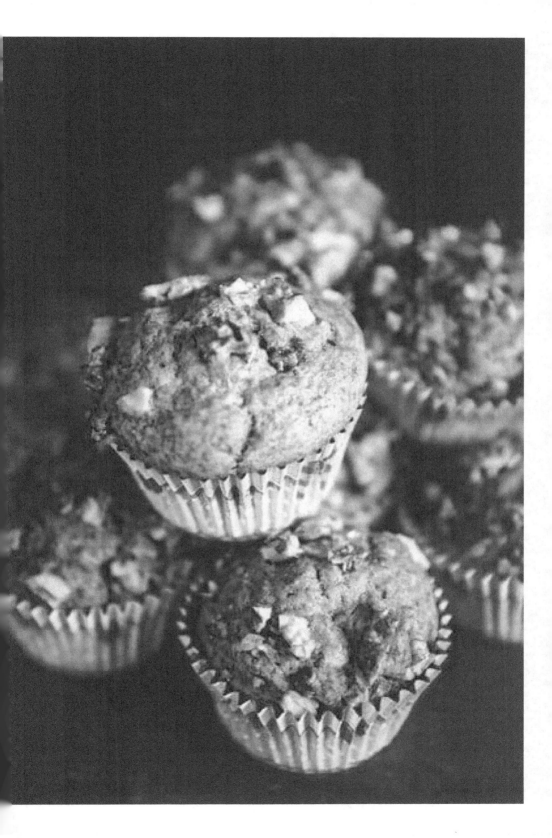

Anti-Inflammatory Porridge

3 Servings

Preparation Time: 15 minutes

Ingredients

- ¼ cup Walnuts, chopped and toasted
- 2 tablespoons hemp seeds, toasted
- 2 tablespoons chia seeds
- 1 cup Almond milk, unsweetened
- ¼ cup Coconut milk, unsweetened
- ¼ cup Coconut, shredded and toasted
- ¼ cup Almond butter
- 1 tablespoon Coconut oil, melted
- ½ teaspoon turmeric powder
- 1 teaspoon bee pollen
- A pinch of Black pepper

Directions

- Heat up a pot with the Almond and Coconut milk over medium heat, add the walnuts, hemp seeds, chia seeds, coconut, turmeric, black pepper and the bee pollen, stir, and cook for 5 minutes.

- Take off heat, add the Coconut oil and the Almond butter, stir and let sit for 10 minutes, then divide into 2 bowls and serve.

Cucumber Smoothie

3 Servings

Preparation Time: 10 minutes

Ingredients

- 2 cups kale, torn
- 1 cup brewed green tea
- 1 cup Pineapple chunks
- 1 cup cucumber, peeled and chopped
- ½ cup Mango chunks, frozen
- ½ Banana, peeled
- 1 teaspoon ground Ginger
- ¼ teaspoon ground turmeric
- 3 mint leaves, chopped
- 1 tablespoon chia seeds
- 4 ice cubes
- 1 scoop protein powder

Directions

- In your food processor, mix the kale with the green tea, Pineapple, cucumber, mango, Banana, Ginger, turmeric, mint, protein powder and ice.
- Pulse well, then add the chia seeds. Stir, divide into 2 glasses and serve.

Raspberry and Avocado Smoothie

1 Serving

Preparation Time: 10 minutes

Ingredients

- 1 Avocado, pitted and peeled
- ¾ cup Raspberry juice
- ¾ cup Orange juice
- ½ cup Raspberries

Directions

- In your food processor, mix the avocado with the raspberry juice, orange juice and raspberries.
- Pulse well, divide into 2 glasses and serve.

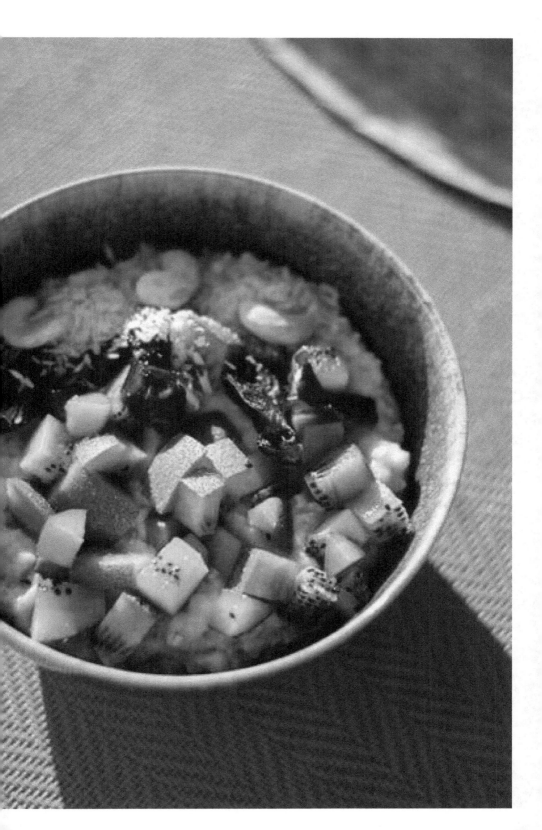

Gingerbread Oatmeal

6 Servings

Preparation Time: 25 minutes

Ingredients

- 1 cup steel cut Oats
- 4 cups water
- ¼ teaspoon ground Coriander
- 1½ tablespoons ground Cinnamon
- ¼ teaspoon ground cloves
- ¼ teaspoon fresh grated ginger
- ¼ teaspoon ground allspice
- ¼ teaspoon ground Cardamom
- A pinch of ground Nutmeg

Directions

- Heat up a pan with the water over medium-high heat, add the Oats and stir.

- Add the coriander, cinnamon, cloves, ginger, allspice, cardamom and nutmeg, stir, cook for 15 minutes, divide into bowls and serve.

Rhubarb Vanilla Muffins

10 Servings

Preparation Time: 35 minutes

Ingredients

- ½ cup Almond meal
- 2 tablespoons crystallized ginger
- ¼ cup Coconut sugar
- 1 tablespoon linseed meal
- ½ cup buckwheat flour
- ¼ cup brown rice flour
- 2 tablespoons powdered arrowroot
- 2 teaspoons gluten-free baking powder
- ½ teaspoon fresh grated ginger
- ½ teaspoon ground cinnamon
- 1 cup rhubarb, sliced
- 1 apple, cored, peeled and chopped
- 1/3 cup Almond milk, unsweetened
- ¼ cup Olive oil

- 1 free-range egg

- 1 teaspoon vanilla extract

Directions

- In a bowl, mix the Almond meal with the crystallized ginger, sugar, linseed meal, buckwheat flour, rice flour, and arrowroot powder, grated ginger, baking powder and cinnamon and stir.
- In another bowl, mix the rhubarb with the apple, Almond milk, oil, egg and vanilla and stir well.
- Combine the 2 mixtures, stir well, and divide into a lined muffin tray. Place in the oven at 350° and bake for 25 minutes.
- Serve the muffins for breakfast.

Winter Fruit Salad

6 Servings

Preparation Time: 10 minutes

Ingredients

- 4 Persimmons, cubed

- 4 Pears, cubed

- 1 cup grapes, halved

- 1 cup apples, peeled, cored and cubed

- ¾ cup pecans, halved

- 1 tablespoon Olive oil

- 1 tablespoon peanut oil

- 1 tablespoon pomegranate flavored vinegar

- 2 tablespoons agave nectar

Directions

- In a mixing bowl, mix the persimmons with the pears, grapes, apples and pecans.

38

- In another bowl, mix the Olive oil with the peanut oil, vinegar and agave nectar.
- Whisk well, then pour over the salad, toss and serve for breakfast.

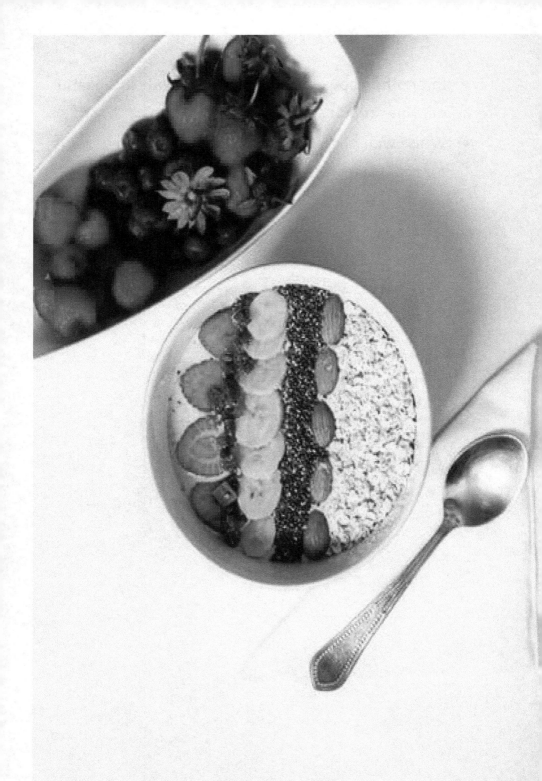

Cocoa Buckwheat Granola

4 Servings

Preparation Time: 55 minutes

Ingredients

- 2 cups Oats
- 1 cup buckwheat
- 1 cup Sunflower seeds
- 1 cup Pumpkin seeds
- 1½ cups Dates, pitted and chopped
- 1 cup Apple puree
- 6 tablespoons Coconut oil
- 5 tablespoons cocoa powder
- 1 teaspoon fresh grated ginger

Directions

- In a large bowl, mix the Oats with the buckwheat, sunflower seeds, pumpkin seeds, dates, Apple puree, oil, cocoa powder, and ginger, then stir really well.

- Spread on a lined baking sheet, press well and place in the oven at 360 degrees ° for 45 minutes.
- Leave the granola to cool down, slice and serve for breakfast.

DRINKS & SMOOTHIES

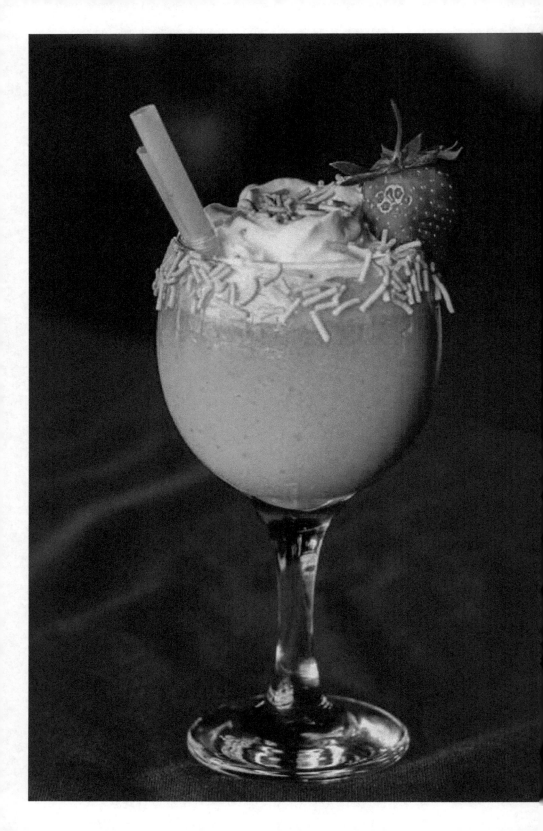

Spinach and Radish Smoothie

6 Servings

Preparation time: 5 minutes

Ingredients

- 1 cup of Coconut milk
- ½ Lemon
- 1 tablespoon Walnuts, chopped
- 1 cup Radish, chopped
- 2 cups Spinach, chopped

Directions

- Put all the ingredients in the blender.
- Blend the smoothie until smooth, and then serve.

Apple Smoothie

6 Servings

Preparation time: 5 minutes

Ingredients

- 1 cup of Water
- 1 cup Apples, chopped
- 1 cup Apricots, chopped

Directions

- Blend the apricots with apples and blend until smooth.
- Add water and stir the smoothie, and then serve.

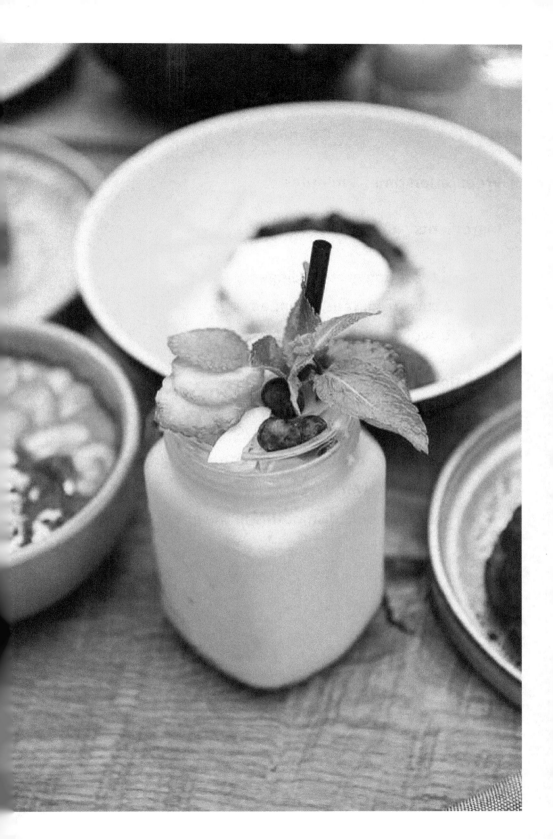

Tomato Smoothie

6 Servings

Preparation time: 5 minutes

Ingredients

- ½ teaspoon ground Ginger
- 2 cups Tomatoes, chopped
- 1 Avocado, chopped

Directions

- Blend the tomatoes with avocado.
- When the mixture is smooth, add ground ginger and carefully mix.
- Pour the cooked smoothie in the glasses and serve.

Mango and Cherries Smoothie

6 Servings

Preparation time: 5 minutes

Ingredients

- 1 cup of Water
- 1 teaspoon Dried mint
- 1 Orange, peeled, chopped
- 1 cup Cherries, pitted
- 1 Mango, peeled, chopped

Directions

- Put all the ingredients in the blender.
- Blend the smoothie until it is smooth and pour in the glasses, and then serve.

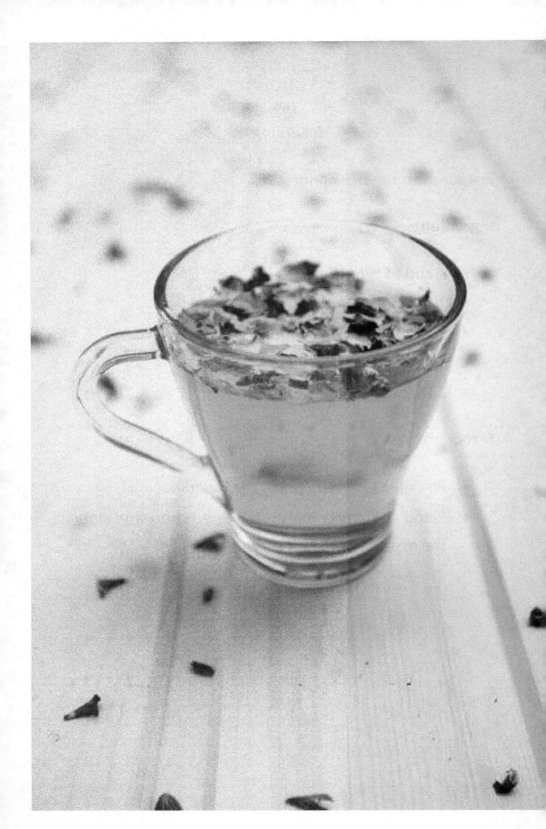

Cayenne Pepper Smoothie

6 Servings

Preparation time: 5 minutes

Ingredients

- ½ cup fresh Spinach, chopped
- 1 cup of Water
- 2 tablespoons Coconut shred
- 1 cup of Coconut milk
- 1 teaspoon Cayenne pepper
- 1 Avocado, chopped

Directions

- Blend the cayenne pepper, avocado, spinach, water, coconut shred, and coconut milk until smooth and serve.

Turmeric Smoothie

4 Servings

Preparation time: 5 minutes

Ingredients

- 2 Bananas, chopped
- 1 tablespoon fresh Lemon juice
- 1 tablespoon ground Turmeric
- 1 cup of Coconut milk

Directions

- Put all the ingredients in the blender.
- Blend the smoothie well, and then serve.

Herbal Tea

6 Servings

Preparation time: 25 minutes

Ingredients

- 6 cups of Water
- 2 tablespoons Herbal tea
- 1 Orange, sliced

Directions

- Bring the water to boil.
- Then remove it from the oven and add herbal tea and oranges.
- Leave the tea for 15 minutes and then serve.

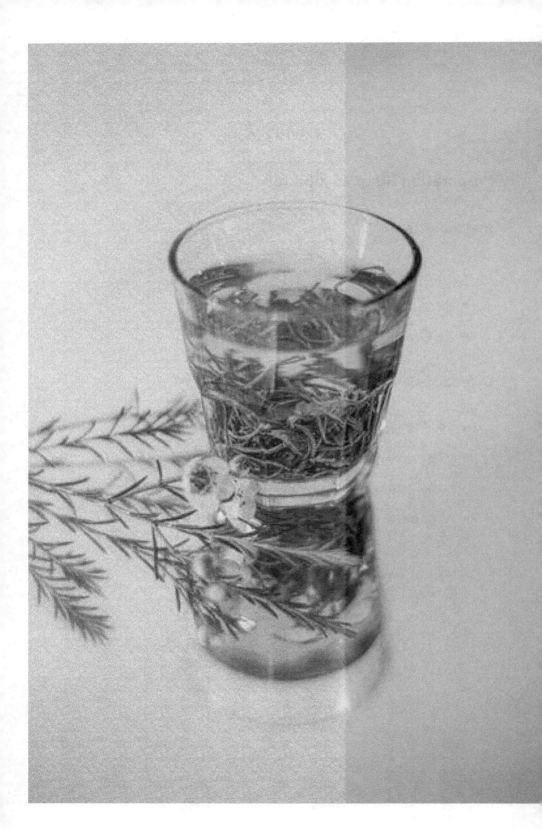

Lemonade

6 Servings

Preparation time: 5 minutes

Ingredients

- 2 tablespoons Mint
- Ice cubes
- 6 cups of Water
- 2 Lemons, sliced

Directions

- Mix the water with lemon and mint.
- Blend the mixture gently.
- Pour it in the glasses and add ice cubes and then serve.

LUNCH

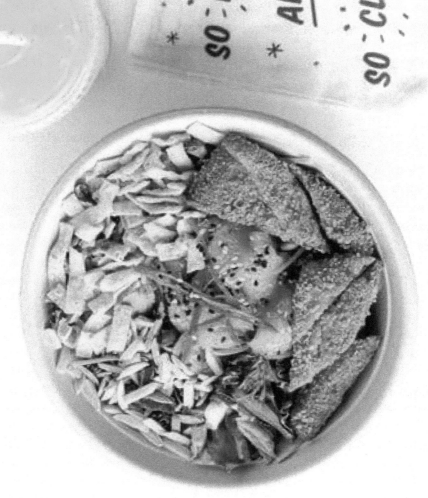

Spicy Eggplant Stew

4 Servings

Preparation Time: 35 minutes

Ingredients

- ½ teaspoon Cumin seeds
- 1 tablespoon coriander seeds
- ½ teaspoon mustard seeds
- 5 eggplants, cubed
- 2 tablespoons coconut, shredded, unsweetened
- 1 teaspoon fresh grated Ginger
- 2 Garlic cloves, minced
- 1 green chili pepper, chopped
- A pinch of cayenne pepper
- A pinch of ground cinnamon
- ½ teaspoon ground cardamom
- ½ teaspoon ground turmeric
- A pinch of salt and black pepper

- 1 teaspoon lime juice

- 1 cup vegetable stock

- 1 tablespoon chopped Parsley

Directions

- Heat up a pan over medium-high heat and add the cumin, coriander, mustard seeds, coconut, ginger, garlic, chili pepper, cayenne, cinnamon, cardamom, turmeric, salt and pepper.
- Stir and cook for 5-6 minutes. Transfer to a food processor and pulse.
- Transfer to a pot and heat up over medium heat. Add the stock, the eggplant, lime juice and the parsley.
- Mix and cook over medium heat for 30 minutes. Divide into bowls and serve.

Beans and Cauliflower Stew

6 Servings

Preparation Time: 1 hour 10 minutes

Ingredients

- 1 cup black beans, soaked for 12 hours and drained
- 4 Garlic cloves, minced
- 1 yellow onion, chopped
- ½ teaspoon garam masala
- 1-inch fresh grated ginger
- ½ teaspoon ground coriander
- ½ teaspoon cayenne pepper
- 1 teaspoon ground turmeric
- 2 cups unsweetened Coconut shredded
- 2 Tomatoes, pureed
- 1 ½ cups cauliflower florets
- 2 cups veggie stock
- A pinch of salt and black pepper
- 1 teaspoon Olive oil
- ½ teaspoon Cumin seeds

Directions

- Heat up a pot with the oil over medium heat. Add cumin, onion, ginger and garlic, stir and cook for 5 minutes.
- Add the beans, coriander, cayenne pepper, turmeric, coconut, Tomatoes, cauliflower, salt, pepper and stock.
- Stir, cover the pot, cook over medium heat for 1 hour, divide into bowls and serve.

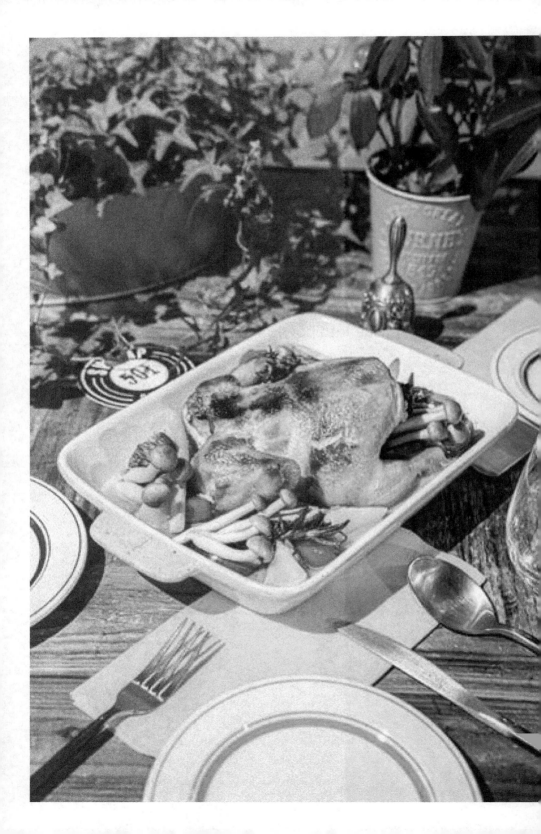

Squash and Chickpea Stew

6 Servings

Preparation Time: 1 hour 10 minutes

Ingredients

- 2 cups chickpeas, soaked overnight and drained
- 2 cups veggie stock
- 1 butternut squash, cubed
- 1 teaspoon Olive oil
- ½ cup red onion, chopped
- ½ teaspoon Cumin seeds
- 4 Garlic cloves minced
- 1 green chili, chopped
- ½ inch fresh grated ginger
- ½ teaspoon garam masala
- ¼ teaspoon ground turmeric
- 1 teaspoon lime juice
- 2 Tomatoes chopped
- A pinch of salt and black pepper
- A pinch of cayenne pepper

- 1 cup spinach
- 1 tablespoon chopped cilantro

Directions

- Heat up a pot with the oil over medium heat.
- Add cumin, chili, garlic, ginger and onions, stir and sauté them for 5 minutes. Add turmeric, garam masala, lime juice, spinach, tomato, stir and cook for 5 minutes.
- Add chickpeas, stock, salt, pepper, cayenne, squash, stir, simmer over medium heat for 45 minutes.
- Add the spinach and the cilantro, mix and cook for 5 minutes more, then divide into bowls and serve.

Black Beans Chili

6 Servings

Preparation Time: 1 hour 25 minutes

Ingredients

- 1 red bell pepper, chopped
- 2 teaspoons Olive oil
- 2 yellow onions, chopped
- 6 Garlic cloves, minced
- 1 green bell pepper, chopped
- 24 ounces canned black beans, drained
- 6 cups veggie stock
- 1 tablespoon cocoa powder
- 2 tablespoons chili powder, mild
- 2 teaspoons ground Cumin
- ½ teaspoon chipotle powder
- 2 teaspoons smoked paprika
- 30 ounces canned Tomatoes, chopped
- 1/3 cup quinoa
- 1½ cups corn
- A pinch of salt and black pepper

Directions

- Heat up a pot with the oil over medium heat. Add onions, stir and cook them for 5 minutes.
- Add red peppers, green bell peppers, garlic, stock, beans, cocoa powder, chili powder, cumin, chipotle powder, paprika and Tomatoes.
- Stir everything together, cover and cook over medium heat for about 50 minutes.
- Add quinoa, corn, salt and pepper, stir, cook for 10-15 minutes more, then divide into bowls and serve.

Barley Soup with Mushrooms

6 Servings

Preparation Time: 1 hour 20 minutes

Ingredients

- 2 yellow onions, chopped
- ¼ cup pearl barley
- 4 cups veggie stock
- 6 ounces brown mushrooms, halved
- A pinch of salt and black pepper
- 3 Garlic cloves, minced
- 2 teaspoons chopped thyme
- 12 ounces cabbage, shredded
- ½ teaspoon smoked paprika
- ½ teaspoon hot paprika
- 4 cups Water
- 16 ounces canned black beans, drained and rinsed
- 1 tablespoon lemon juice

Directions

- In a pot, mix stock with the barley. Stir, bring to a simmer over medium heat and cook for 30 minutes.
- Add mushrooms, cabbage, smoked paprika, hot paprika, garlic, onions, salt, pepper, thyme, beans, lemon juice and water.
- Stir, cover the pot, and cook over medium heat for 40 minutes more. Ladle into bowls and serve.

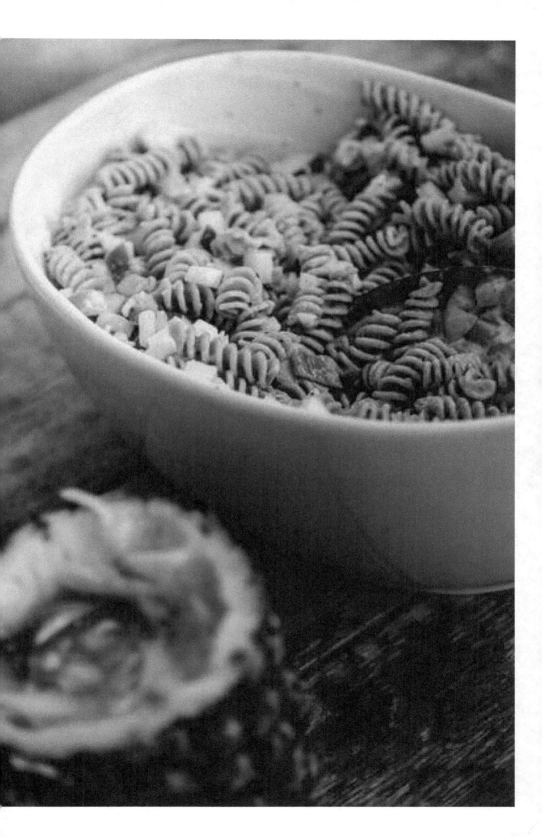

Spicy Chicken and Zucchini Meatballs

6 Servings

Preparation Time: 20 minutes

Ingredients

- 1 cup shredded zucchini
- 2 pounds ground Chicken
- 2 tablespoons harissa
- 1 Garlic clove, minced
- ¼ cup chopped green onions
- 1 egg
- 2 tablespoons balsamic vinegar
- 1 tablespoon maple syrup
- A pinch of salt and black pepper

Directions

- In a bowl, mix Chicken with zucchini, green onions, egg, Garlic clove, harissa, balsamic vinegar, salt, pepper and maple syrup, stir well and shape into medium meatballs.

- Heat up a pan with the oil over medium heat, add the meatballs and cook them for 5 minutes on each side.
- Divide between plates and serve for lunch with a side salad.

Crispy Cod

2 Servings

Preparation Time: 25 minutes

Ingredients

- 1 egg white
- ½ cup red quinoa, already cooked
- 2 teaspoons whole wheat flour
- 4 teaspoons lemon juice
- ½ teaspoon smoked paprika
- 3 teaspoons Olive oil
- 2 medium black cod fillets, skinless and boneless
- 1 red plum, pitted and chopped
- 2 teaspoons raw honey
- ¼ teaspoon black peppercorns, crushed
- 2 teaspoons Parsley
- ¼ cup Water

Directions

- In a bowl, whisk together 1 teaspoon lemon juice with egg white, flour and ¼ teaspoon paprika.
- Add quinoa in a bowl and mix it with 1/3 of egg white mix. Add the fish into the bowl with the remaining egg white mix, toss to coat, then dip the fish in quinoa mix and also toss to coat.
- Heat up a pan with 1 teaspoon oil over medium heat and add peppercorns, honey and plum.
- Stir, bring to a simmer and cook for 1 minute. Add the rest of the lemon juice, the rest of the paprika and the water to the pan, stir well and simmer for 5 minutes.
- Add parsley, stir, take the sauce off the heat and set aside for now.
- Heat up a pan with the rest of the Olive oil over medium heat; add the coated fish cook for 3 minutes.
- Move the fish to a lined sheet tray and bake in the oven at 400 degrees ° for 10 minutes more.
- Divide between plates, drizzle the plums sauce all over and serve.

Greek Sea Bass Mix

6 Servings

Preparation Time: 32 minutes

Ingredients

- 2 sea bass fillets, boneless
- 1 Garlic clove, minced
- 5 cherry Tomatoes, halved
- 1 tablespoon chopped Parsley
- 2 shallots, chopped
- Juice of ½ lemon
- 1 tablespoon Olive oil
- 8 ounces baby spinach
- Cooking spray

Directions

- Grease a baking dish with cooking oil, then add the fish, Tomatoes, Parsley and garlic.

- Drizzle the lemon juice over the fish, cover the dish and place it in the oven at 350 degrees F. Bake for 15 minutes and then divide between plates.
- Heat up a pan with the Olive oil over medium heat, add shallot, stir and cook for 1 minute.
- Add spinach, stir, cook for 5 minutes more, add to the plate with the fish and serve.

Thyme Carrots

6 Servings

Preparation Time: 50 minutes

Ingredients

- 8 Carrots, peeled
- 1 tablespoon dried thyme
- 2 tablespoons lemon juice
- 2 tablespoons Olive oil

Directions

- In the shallow bowl, mix dried thyme with lemon juice and Olive oil.

- Then place the Carrots in the tray and sprinkle with thyme mixture.

- Bake the Carrot at 360° for 40 minutes.

DINNER

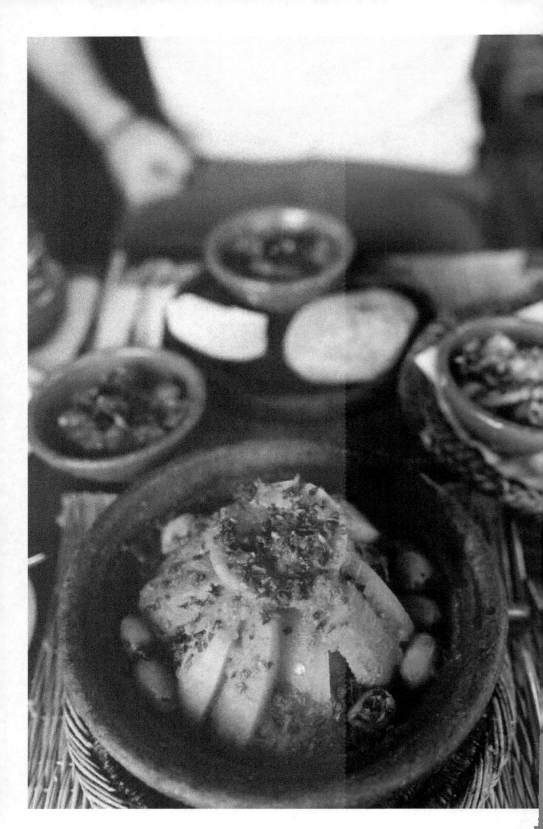

Chickpeas Spread

2 Servings

Preparation Time: 10 minuets

Ingredients

- 1 cup Chickpeas, cooked
- 1 tablespoon Tahini paste
- 2 tablespoons Lemon juice
- ¼ cup Olive oil

Directions

- Add all ingredients in the food processor.
- Blend the mixture until smooth.
- Transfer it in the serving bowl.

Baked Cremini Mushrooms

5 Servings

Preparation Time: 40 minutes

Ingredients

- 3 cups Cremini Mushrooms
- ¼ cup plain Yogurt
- ¼ cup fresh Parsley, chopped
- 1 teaspoon minced Garlic
- 1 teaspoon ground Turmeric
- 1 tablespoon Olive oil

Directions

- Mix cremini mushrooms with plain yogurt, parsley, and all remaining ingredients.
- Add the mixture in the tray and bake at 350° for 30 minutes.

Bean Spread

4 Servings

Preparation Time: 10 minutes

Ingredients

- 2 cups red Kidney beans, boiled
- 1 teaspoon ground Nutmeg
- 1 teaspoon Cayenne pepper
- 3 tablespoons plain Yogurt
- 1 tablespoon fresh Cilantro, chopped

Directions

- Blend the red kidney beans until you get a smooth paste.
- Then mix the beans with plain yogurt, ground nutmeg, cayenne pepper, and cilantro.
- Carefully mix the spread.

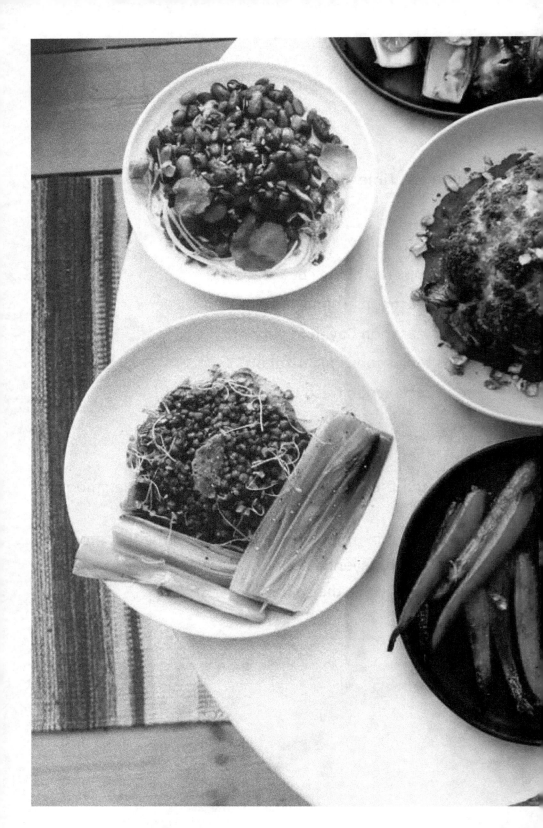

Turmeric Salmon

6 Servings

Preparation Time: 20 minutes

Ingredients

- 1-pound Salmon fillet, chopped
- 1 teaspoon ground Turmeric
- 1 teaspoon ground Ginger
- 2 tablespoons Olive oil

Directions

- Mix Salmon fillet with ground turmeric and ground Ginger.
- Preheat the Olive oil in the pan. Add salmon.
- Roast the fish on medium heat for 4 minutes per side.

Salmon Meatballs

5 Servings

Preparation Time: 22 minutes

Ingredients

- 1-pound Salmon fillet, minced
- 1 teaspoon ground coriander
- 1 tablespoon Olive oil
- 1 tablespoon minced Garlic
- 2 tablespoons Almond flour

Directions

- Mix Salmon fillet with minced garlic, Almond flour, and ground coriander.
- Make the meatballs.
- Preheat the pan well, add Olive oil.
- Add the Salmon meatballs in the hot oil and roast them for 3 minutes per side.

Spinach Chicken

6 Servings

Preparation Time: 50 minutes

Ingredients

- 1-pound Chicken breast, skinless, boneless, chopped
- 2 cups spinach, chopped
- 1 teaspoon minced Ginger
- 1 teaspoon chili pepper
- 1 cup of Coconut milk

Directions

- Add all ingredients in the saucepan and carefully mix.
- Close the lid and simmer the meal on medium-low heat for 40 minutes.
- Serve the cooked meal in the bowls.

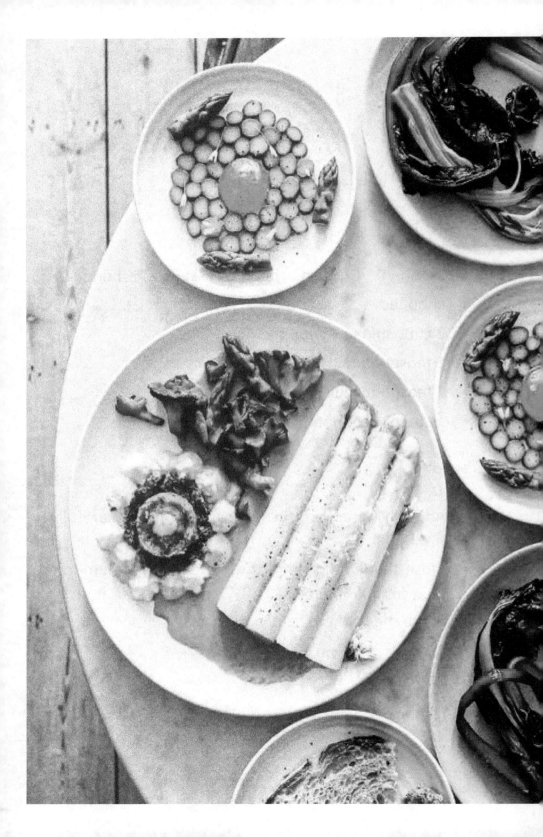

Chicken with Strawberries

6 Servings

Preparation Time: 45 minutes

Ingredients

- 1-pound Chicken breast, skinless, boneless, chopped
- 1 cup strawberries, chopped
- 1 cup of Water
- 1 teaspoon dried mint
- 1 teaspoon chili powder
- 1 tablespoon Olive oil

Directions

- Roast the Chicken breast with Olive oil for 2 minutes per side.
- Then add strawberries, water, dried mint, and chili powder.
- Close the lid and cook the meal on medium heat for 30 minutes.

Curry Chicken

6 Servings

Preparation Time: 36 minutes

Ingredients

- 1-pound Chicken breast, skinless, boneless, chopped
- 1 tablespoon curry paste
- ½ cup of Coconut milk
- 1 teaspoon lemongrass, chopped
- 1 teaspoon Olive oil

Directions

- Mix the curry paste with Coconut milk and lemongrass.
- Roast the Chicken with Olive oil for 3 minutes per side.
- Then add Coconut milk mixture and stir the meal.
- Close the lid and cook the Chicken on medium heat for 20 minutes.

SALADS

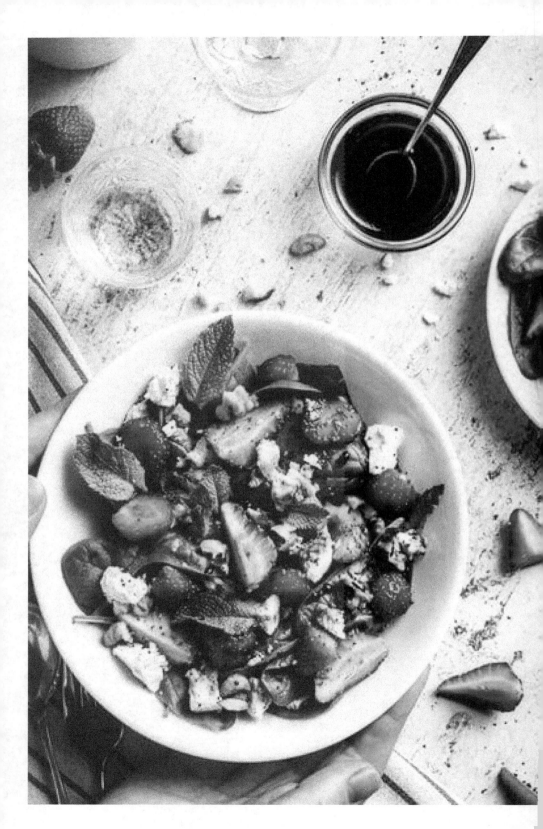

Salmon Salad

6 Servings

Preparation Time: 10 minutes

Ingredients

- 1-pound Salmon fillet, boiled
- 1 white Onion, diced
- 1 cup Lettuce, chopped
- 1 cup Spinach, chopped
- 1 tablespoon Lemon juice
- 1 teaspoon Olive oil
- 1 teaspoon ground Paprika

Directions

- Put salmon fillet, onion, lettuce, spinach, and ground paprika, in the salad bowl. Shake the mixture.
- Then sprinkle the salad with olive oil and lemon juice.

Peach Salad

6 Servings

Preparation Time: 5 minutes

Ingredients

- 1 cup Lettuce, chopped
- 1 tablespoon Olive oil
- 2 cups Peaches, chopped
- 12 oz cod Fillet, boiled, chopped
- 1 tablespoon Lime juice
- 1 tablespoon Scallions, chopped
- 1 teaspoon minced Garlic

Directions

- Mix lettuce with scallions, minced garlic, peaches, and cod fillet.
- Put the salad in the serving plates and sprinkle it with lime juice and olive oil.

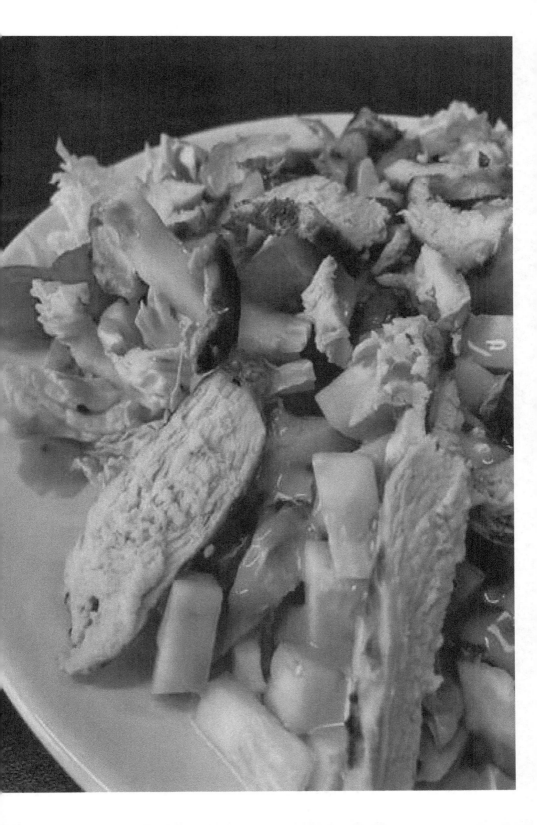

Pineapple Salad

6 Servings

Preparation Time: 10 minutes

Ingredients

- 10 oz Pineapple, chopped
- 1 tablespoon Coconut cream
- 1 teaspoon Lemon juice
- 1 tablespoon Coconut shred
- 1 Mango, chopped

Directions

- Mix pineapple with mango, and coconut shred.
- Then sprinkle the salad with coconut cream and lemon juice.

Chives Salad

6 Servings

Preparation Time: 5 minutes

Ingredients

- 4 Eggs, boiled, peeled, chopped
- 1 Cucumber, chopped
- ¼ cup Coconut cream
- 1 teaspoon ground Black pepper
- 8 oz Chives, chopped

Directions

- Mix chives with eggs, cucumber, and ground black pepper.
- Add coconut cream.
- Carefully mix the salad.

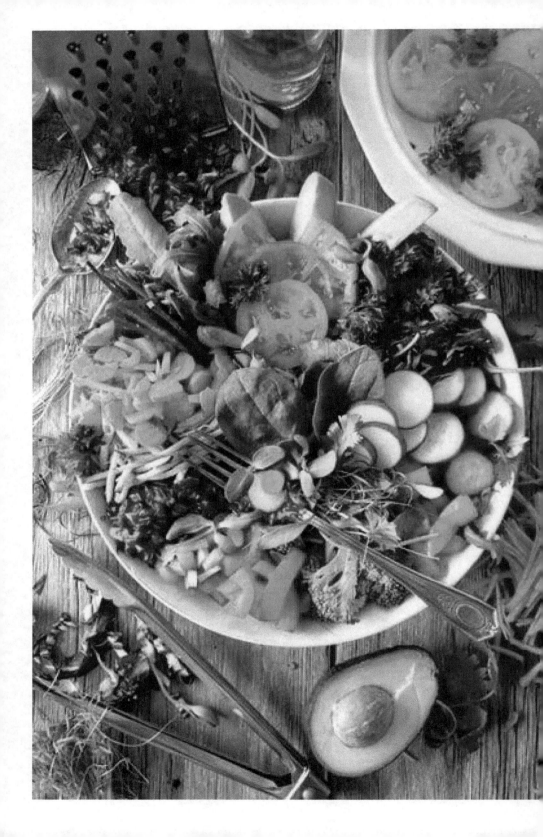

Slaw

6 Servings

Preparation Time: 10 minutes

Ingredients

- 1 Carrot, grated
- 1 tablespoon Olive oil
- 2 tablespoons Lemon juice
- ½ teaspoon ground Clove
- 2 cups white Cabbage, shredded
- 1 Apple, chopped

Directions

- Put all ingredients in the salad bowl and carefully mix.
- Leave the salad for at least 5 minutes to rest before serving.

Apple Salad

6 Servings

Preparation Time: 5 minutes

Ingredients

- 2 Apples, chopped
- 1 tablespoon raw Honey
- ½ teaspoon ground Cinnamon
- 1 Carambola, chopped
- 2 oz Raisins, chopped
- 1 tablespoon Lemon juice

Directions

- Mix apples with raisins and carambola.
- Add ground cinnamon, raw honey, and lemon juice.
- Stir the salad well.

Spinach Salad

6 Servings

Preparation Time: 5 minutes

Ingredients

- 2 cups Spinach, chopped
- 1 cup Tomatoes, chopped
- 1 tablespoon Olive oil
- ¼ teaspoon ground Clove
- 3 tablespoons Lemon juice

Directions

- Mix spinach with lemon juice, tomatoes, and olive oil.
- Top the salad with ground clove and put it in the serving plates.

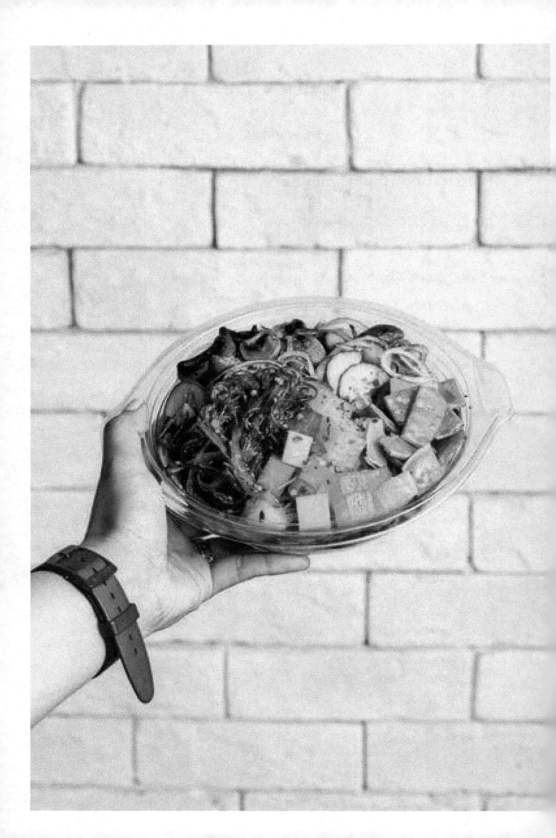

Mint Salad

6 Servings

Preparation Time: 10 minutes

Ingredients

- 1 tablespoon Fresh mint, chopped
- 3 cups green Cabbage, shredded
- 1 tablespoon Lemon juice
- 1 tablespoon Olive oil
- 1 tablespoon Cranberries
- 3 oz Sallions, chopped

Directions

- Put all ingredients in the salad bowl.
- Gently shake the salad.

DESSERTS

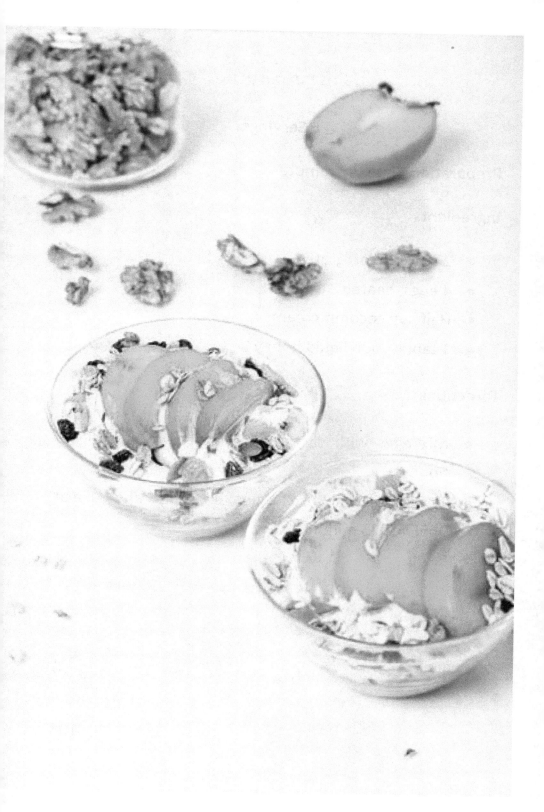

Carrot Soufflé

6 Servings

Preparation Time: 45 minutes

Ingredients

- 2 cups carrot, grated.
- 4 eggs, beaten.
- Half cup coconut cream
- 1 tablespoon liquid honey

Directions

- Mix eggs with carrot, coconut cream, and liquid honey.
- Transfer the mixture in the baking cups and bake at 365F for 25 minutes.

Baked Bananas

8 Servings

Preparation Time: 35 minutes

Ingredients

- 6 bananas cut in halves.
- 1 teaspoon ground cinnamon
- 1 teaspoon vanilla extract
- 1 tablespoon almond butter

Directions

- Rub the banana halves with ground cinnamon, vanilla extract, and almond butter.
- Put the bananas in the tray and bake at 365F for 15 minutes.

Pomegranate Pudding

6 Servings

Preparation Time: 40 minutes

Ingredients

- 1 cup oatmeal
- 2 cups of coconut milk
- 3 almond butter
- Half cup pomegranate seeds.

Directions

- Bring the coconut milk to a boil.
- Add oatmeal and almond butter.
- Simmer the mixture for 5 minutes.
- Then remove it from the heat, **add pomegranate seeds and mix well.**
- Transfer the pudding in the serving bowls.

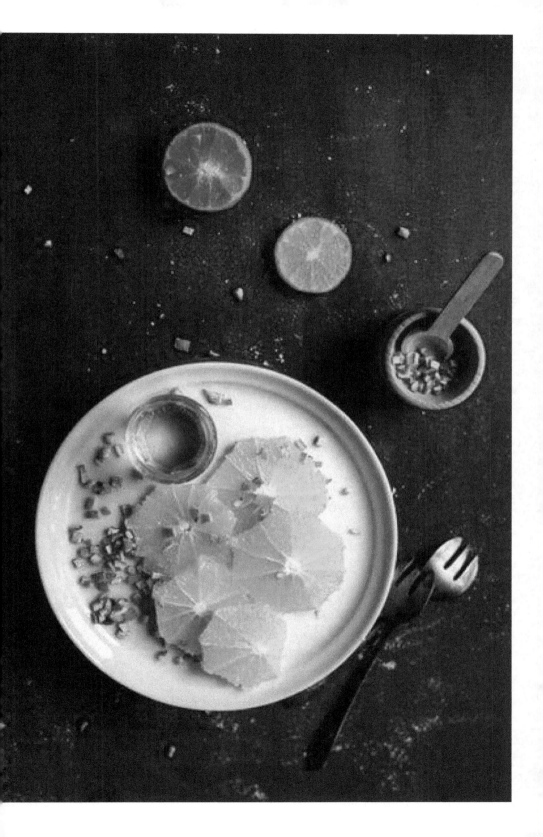

Mango Pudding

4 Servings

Preparation Time: 20 minutes

Ingredients

- 1 mango, peeled, blended.
- 1 cup plain yogurt
- 3 ounces chia seeds
- 1 teaspoon fresh mint

Directions

- Mix plain yogurt with chia seeds and put in the serving glasses.
- Top the yogurt with fresh mint and blended mango.

Matcha Pudding

6 Servings

Preparation Time: 30 minutes

Ingredients

- 1 teaspoon matcha powder
- 1 cup coconut cream
- 2 ounces chia seeds
- 1 tablespoon liquid honey

Directions

- Mix matcha powder with coconut cream and bring to boil.
- Then cool the mixture, add chia seeds and liquid honey.
- Mix the pudding well.

Pineapple Sorbet

6 Servings

Preparation Time: 60 minutes

Ingredients

- 2 tbsps of liquid honey
- 1 teaspoon fresh mint
- 2 cups pineapple, chopped.

Directions

- Blend the pineapple until smooth.
- Add liquid honey and mint. Mix the mixture.
- Put the mixture in the silicone molds and freeze for 40 minutes.
- Then remove the mixture from the molds, transfer in the food processor and blend until smooth.
- Put the dessert in the serving bowls.

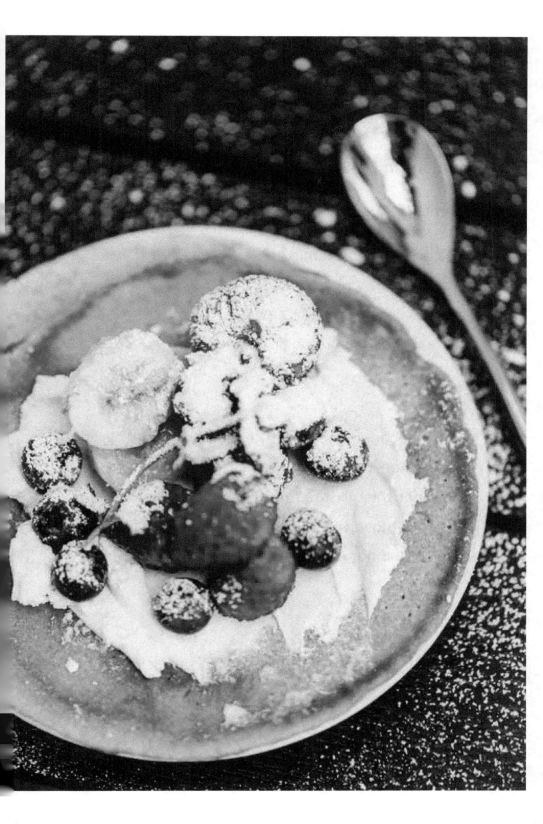

Cinnamon Brown Rice Pudding

6 Servings

Preparation Time: 45 minutes

Ingredients

- 3 cups of coconut milk
- 1 cup of brown rice
- 1 tablespoon liquid honey
- 1 teaspoon cinnamon powder

Directions

- Mix coconut milk with brown rice and ground cinnamon.
- Simmer the mixture for 20 minutes on low heat.
- Then remove the pudding from the heat, cool little, add liquid honey, and mix the pudding well.

Watermelon Cream

8 Servings

Preparation Time: 2 hours and30 minutes

Ingredients

- 1 watermelon peeled and cubed.
- 1 teaspoon vanilla extract
- Half teaspoon cinnamon powder
- 2 mangoes peeled and cubed.

Directions

- In a blender, combine the watermelon with the mango and the other ingredients.
- Pulse well, divide into bowls and keep in the fridge for 2 hours before serving.

CPSIA information can be obtained
at www.ICGtesting.com
Printed in the USA
BVHW010340240521
607866BV00032B/1268

9 781802 938562